I0843702

HOME WORKOUT FOR WEIGHT LOSS IN 10 EASY STEP

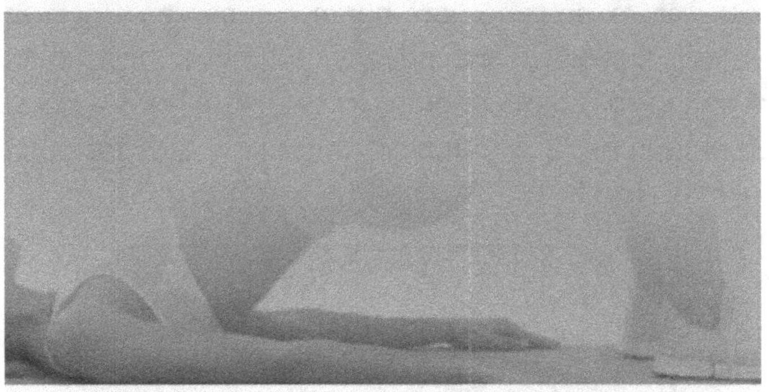

30-Minute Fat-Burning Workout for Beginners

HARRY LANCE

ABSTRACT

Home Workout for Weight Loss: An Effective and Convenient Approach

This abstract explores the growing trend of home-based workouts for achieving weight loss goals. As modern lifestyles become increasingly sedentary, individuals seek practical and time-efficient ways to shed excess pounds without the need for costly gym memberships or specialized equipment. This paper delves into the efficacy of home workout routines, incorporating bodyweight exercises, cardio workouts, and yoga practices. It highlights the benefits of exercising at home, such as increased motivation, flexibility, and privacy. Moreover, the abstract explores the role of technology, including fitness apps and online resources, in enhancing home workouts for optimal weight loss results."

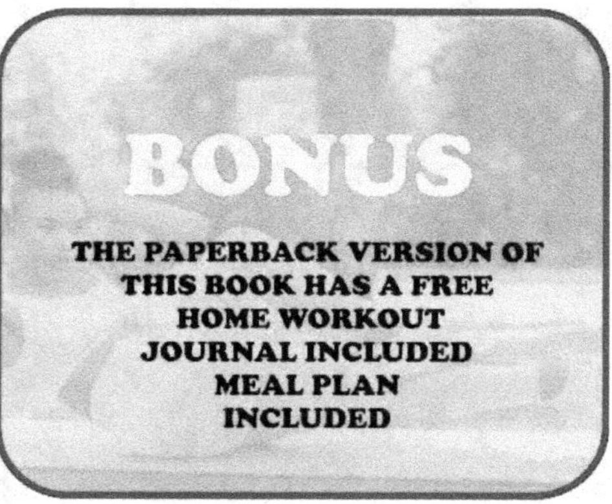

HOME WORKOUT FOR WEIGHT LOSS IN 10 EASY STEP

30-Minute Fat-Burning Workout for Beginners

HARRY LANCE

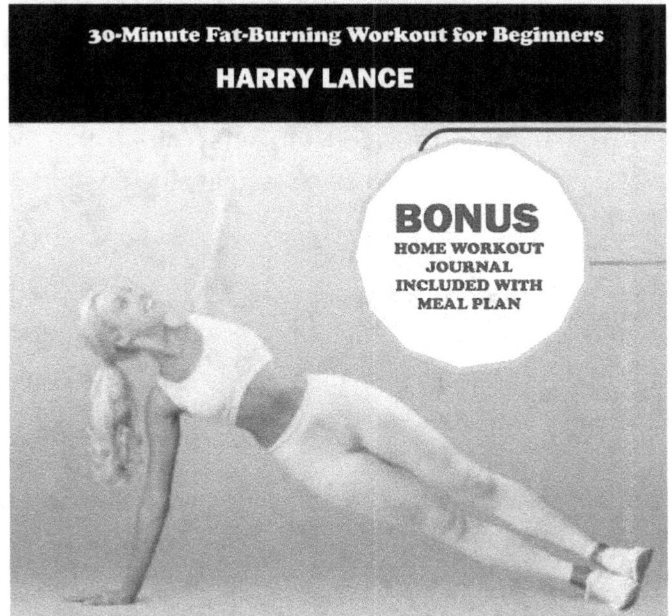

INTRODUCTION

Lucy frequently struggled with fatigue and body dissatisfaction throughout the day. She wanted for a change, a means to get rid of those obstinate extra pounds, and to feel good about herself. She came across a hidden gem one day while perusing her favorite bookstore, "Home Workout For Weight Loss In 10 Easy Steps." She eagerly bought the book and made her way home, intrigued by the prospect of a life-changing voyage.

With the book in her hands, Lucy sat down in her comfortable living room as the sun began to drop. Her excitement rose with each word as she started turning the pages. The manual provided ten easy steps that, when followed, may enable her to lose weight in the comfort of her own home.

The first step was to establish precise, attainable goals. Lucy felt motivated and snatched up a pen and notebook to scribble down her goals and affirmations. She was confident that this time, she would succeed.

The second step emphasized the value of developing a daily exercise schedule. The book included a variety of tasks with detailed directions and visual aids, which Lucy found to be helpful in creating her unique strategy. With renewed vigor, she resolved to schedule some time each day for exercise.

Five emphasized the value of having a support network. Reaching out to her friends and family, Lucy shared her goals and found motivation in their support and encouragement.

As the days passed, Lucy continued to follow her new regimen. Her energy levels increased, and the routines became simpler. She became aware of tiny alterations in her physique and, more crucially, in her attitude.

Adding mindfulness and meditation to her daily practice was the focus of step six. In these peaceful times, Lucy found comfort, which enabled her to keep up her newly acquired good habits and handle her stress.

Step seven emphasized the value of monitoring progress. In order to document her successes, failures, and reflections, Lucy kept a journal. Taking pride in all of her accomplishments, no matter how tiny, served as inspiration.

Step 8 introduced the idea of varying routines to prevent boredom. From yoga to dance workouts, Lucy experimented with a range of exercises and enjoyed the diversity.

Step nine emphasized the importance of relaxation and healing. Lucy discovered how to create a balance between pushing herself and giving herself the time she needed to recuperate by paying attention to her body.

Tenth and last step: accepting the adventure. Lucy understood that this was a journey towards self-discovery, self-love, and personal development rather than merely a means of weight loss.

After several months, Lucy reflected on her accomplishments with admiration. She had finished the book, but more significantly, she had changed for the better. She had lost weight because to her perseverance, commitment, and newly adopted healthy habits, but they had also given her a sense of fulfillment and happiness that she had never known before.

One final time, Lucy closed the book with thankfulness in her heart. She was aware that her life's journey toward a healthier and happier version of herself had only just begun. Hers was a tale of tenacity and victory.

Starting a home workout for weight loss can be a great way to stay active and achieve your fitness goals. Here are 10 easy steps to help you get started:

1.Clear Your Goals: Establish your exercise and weight loss goals. Setting concrete objectives will keep you motivated and concentrated. Consult a physician: It's imperative to speak with your doctor before starting any new exercise program, especially if you have any existing medical ailments or concerns.

2.Make an exercise schedule: Schedule your workouts in advance. Choose the days and times you'll exercise, and make every effort to keep to this routine.

3.Choose Appropriate Workouts: Make your choice of exercises based on your degree of fitness and weight loss objectives.

4 Concentrate on a combination of cardio workouts (such as jogging, jumping jacks, or dancing) and strength training (such as exercises using only your bodyweight, resistance bands, or weights).

5.Always begin your activity with a warm-up to get your body ready for action and lower the risk of injury. Perform a cool-down regimen following each exercise to aid in your body's recovery.

6.Start Slowly: If you've never worked out before or haven't in a while, start with lower-intensity workouts and gradually increase the length and intensity as your fitness level rises.

7.Make a Specific Area for Exercise in Your Home: Create a Special Place for Exercise in Your Home. It can be easier to get in the appropriate frame of mind to exercise if you have a designated location.

8.Use Online tools: There are several online tools that provide guided home workouts for weight loss, such as exercise videos and fitness apps. Make use of these to keep your routine interesting and varied.

9.Drink water before, during, and after your workouts to stay hydrated. Maintaining proper hydration is essential for general health and can aid in weight loss.

10.Track Your Progress: Record your workouts and keep tabs on your development. This can be done via a mobile app, a fitness journal, or even just plain old notes on your phone. Observing your progress over time can motivate you more.

Consistency is important, keep in mind. Your ability to lose weight can be significantly impacted by even brief, frequent workouts. Be patient, pay attention to your body, and remember to enjoy yourself as you progress. Consider reaching out to friends or joining online fitness communities for help and encouragement if you are having trouble or are lacking motivation.

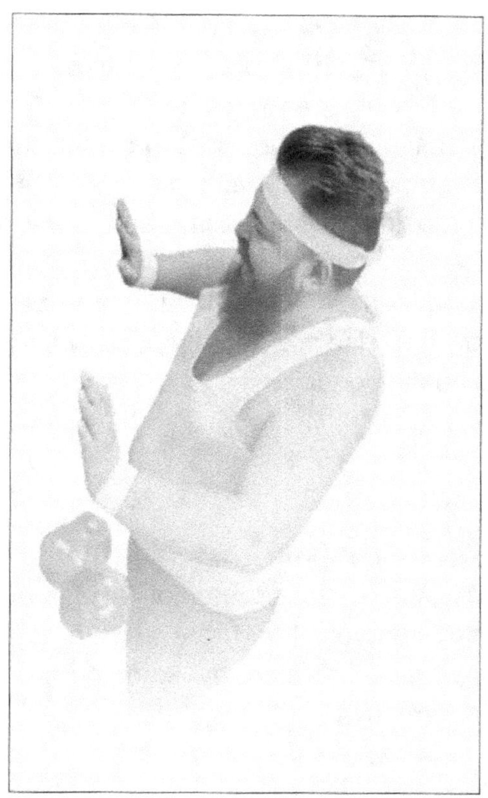

Starting a home workout routine for weight loss can be an effective way to achieve your fitness goals. Remember to combine these exercises with a balanced diet for the best results. Here are 20 home workouts that can help you with weight loss:

Remember to warm up before starting your workout and cool down afterward. Aim for at least 30 minutes of moderate-intensity exercise most days of the week for effective weight loss. As your fitness level improves, consider increasing the intensity and duration of your workouts to challenge your body further. Always listen to your body and consult a healthcare professional before starting a new exercise program, especially if you have any pre-existing health conditions.

1. Jumping Jacks

Jumping jacks are a classic cardiovascular exercise that effectively elevates your heart rate and burns calories. To perform jumping jacks, start by standing with your feet together and arms by your sides.

In one swift motion, jump your feet out to the sides while simultaneously raising your arms overhead. Return to the starting position by jumping your feet back together and lowering your arms. Repeat this movement continuously for a set amount of time or repetitions. Jumping jacks engage multiple muscle groups, including the legs, core, and shoulders. They improve cardiovascular fitness, endurance, and coordination. It's a great warm-up exercise or can be used as part of a high-intensity interval training (HIIT) workout.

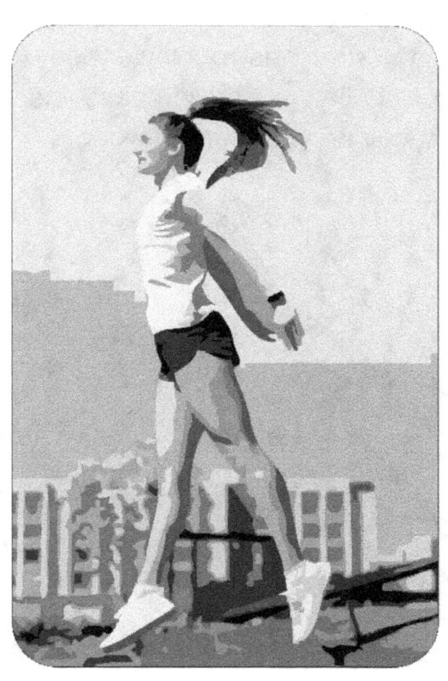

2. High Knees:

Another great cardiovascular workout that strengthens the lower body and core is raising your knees. Stand with your feet hip-width apart to do high knees. Hop on your right foot, lift your left knee as high as you can, then rapidly transition to lifting your right knee while hopping on your left foot. As quickly as you can, keep alternating your knees as you raise them toward your chest.

This workout raises your heart rate, expels calories, and strengthens and stretches your lower body. High knees give an additional challenge and increase the intensity of the workout by requiring your core to work.

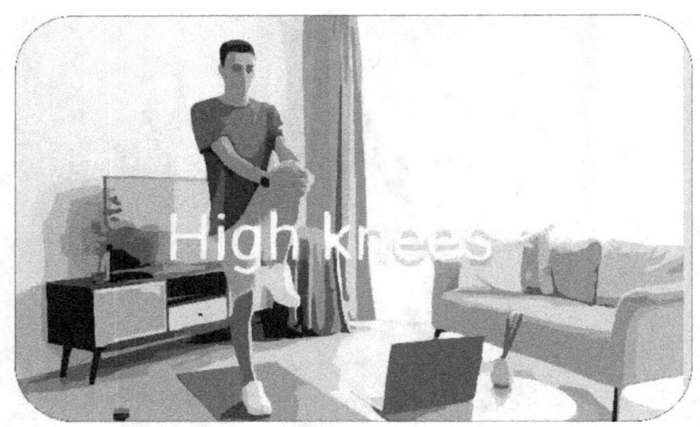

3. Mountain Climbers:

A dynamic, all-body workout that works the core, shoulders, and legs is the mountain climber. Start in a plank position with your hands squarely beneath your shoulders and a straight line extending from your shoulders to your hips. Drive one leg into your chest, then swiftly switch to the other leg as if you were running. Throughout the exercise, keep your core engaged and your hips level.

Mountain climbers provide you a fantastic aerobic workout while also boosting stability and strengthening your core muscles. They can be performed as a stand-alone exercise or included into HIIT programs.

4. Burpees:

Squats, push-ups, and leaps are all included in the high-intensity, full-body exercise known as a burpee. Starting from a standing position with your feet shoulder-width apart, complete a burpee. Kick your feet back into a plank posture after squatting down and placing your hands and feet on the ground. Push-up first, then leap your feet back into a squat and leap up quickly, raising your arms overhead.

Burpees are a fantastic exercise for boosting cardiovascular fitness, burning calories, and developing arm, chest, leg, and core strength. Although they are difficult, they may be altered to accommodate various levels of fitness.

5. Jump Squats:

Jump squats are an efficient plyometric exercise for weight loss and lower body strength because they add an explosive element to regular squats. Start by assuming a shoulder-width position for your feet. Maintaining a straight back and your knees behind your toes, squat down.

Jump up quickly, raising your arms overhead, and softly land back in the squat position. Jump squats exercise the hamstrings, glutes, quadriceps, and calf muscles. The exercise's plyometric nature increases calorie expenditure and enhances power and agility.

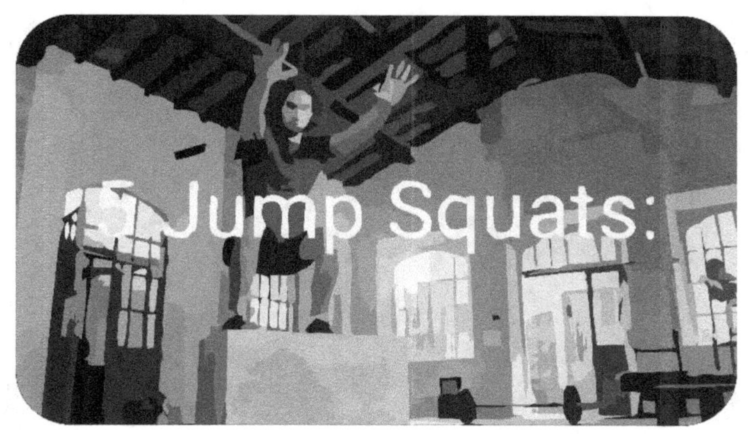

6. Push-Ups:

A popular bodyweight exercise that primarily works the chest, shoulders, and triceps is the push-up. Start off with your hands slightly wider than shoulder width apart in a plank stance. Bending your elbows while maintaining a straight back and an engaged core can help you lower your body to the ground. Return to the beginning posture by exerting pressure via your palms. Push-ups are a great upper body and core exercise that may be changed according to your level of fitness. They aid in increasing total calorie expenditure, muscle tone, and upper body strength.

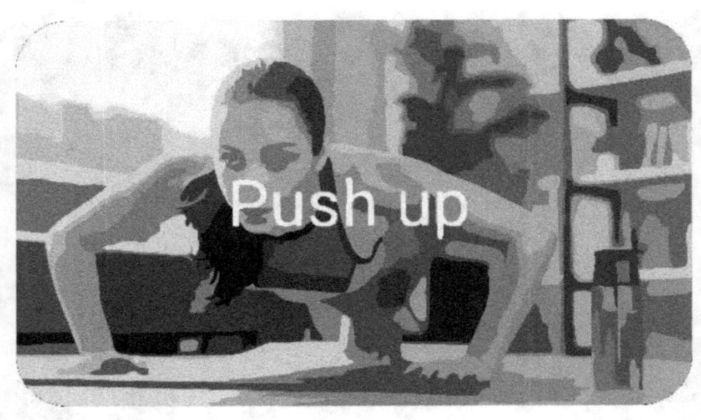

7. Tricep Dips:

Using a solid chair or step will help you perform tricep dips, which focus on the back of your arms. With your fingers pointing forward, sit on the chair's edge with your hands firmly grasping the front edge. Step forward while keeping your hands shoulder-width apart and your arms supporting your weight. Bending your elbows will help you lower your body to the ground, then you should push yourself back up to the beginning position.

The triceps are efficiently isolated and strengthened while the shoulders and core are also worked during tricep dips. In order to prevent stress on the shoulders and wrists, proper form is crucial.

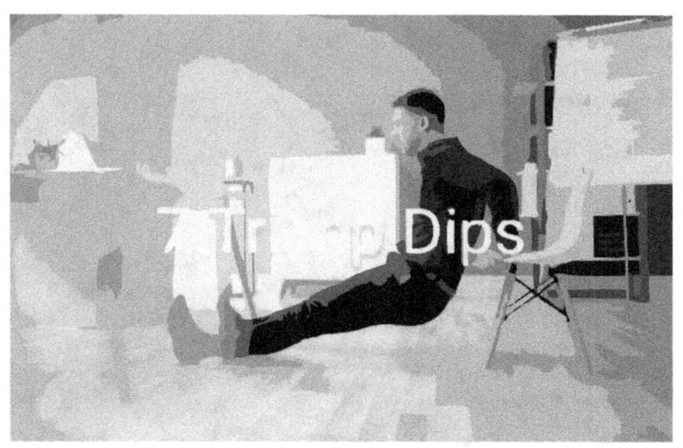

8. Plank:

Keeping a still position is required for the basic core exercise known as the plank. Laying face down, with your elbows just under your shoulders and your forearms resting on the ground, is a good place to start. Using your core and glutes, raise your body in a straight line from the top of your head to your heels. Keep your abs taut and your back flat while holding this position for a predetermined amount of time.

Planks work all of the abdominal muscles, including the rectus, transverse, and obliques.

Additionally, they strengthen the shoulders and correct posture and balance.

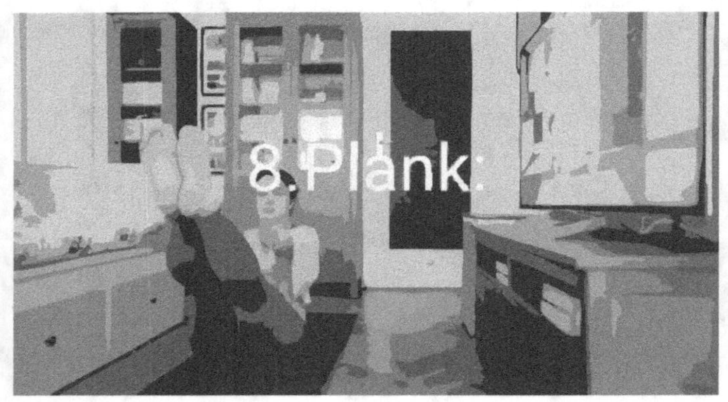

9. Russian Twists:

Russian twists are a useful workout to strengthen the core and target the obliques. Kneel down on the floor with your feet flat on the floor. Lean back slightly while maintaining a straight back and an elevated chest. Twist your torso to the right, then to the left, tapping the floor on either side while you hold your hands together.

Russian twists help define the waistline by working the abdominal muscles. By holding a weight or medicine ball while doing the twists, you can make the exercise more challenging.

10. Bicycle Crunches

A version of the standard crunch that targets the entire abdominal region, including the rectus abdominis and obliques, are bicycle crunches. On your back, elevate your legs with your knees bent 90 degrees.

Place your hands behind your head. Bring your left elbow to your right knee while continuously pedaling your legs as if you were on a bicycle. Then, transition to bringing your right elbow to your left knee while extending your right leg.

Exercises for the core that also work the hip flexors and increase total core stability include bicycle crunches.

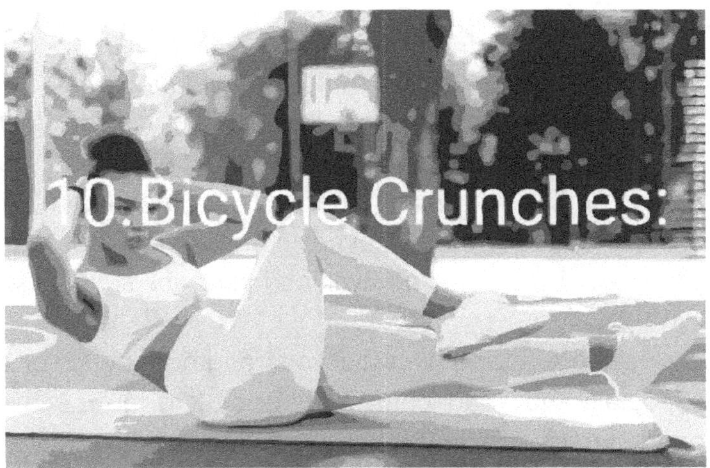

10.   Lunges:

Exercises for the lower body that work the quadriceps, hamstrings, glutes, and calves include lunges. Start by putting your feet together and standing. Step forward with your right foot, lowering your body until your left knee is just above the floor and your right thigh is parallel to the ground. Repeat on the other side, pushing through your right heel to go back to the beginning position.

Exercises like lunges help increase lower body strength, balance, and functional fitness. They can be carried out while carrying dumbbells for increased resistance or using your own bodyweight.

11. Wall Sits:

An isometric exercise that predominantly works the quadriceps is wall sits. Standing with your back against a wall, sit down while keeping your knees bent at a 90-degree angle and your thighs parallel to the floor. For a predetermined period of time, maintain this position with your back flat against the wall and your abs tight.

Wall sits are a great workout to strengthen the lower body, especially the quadriceps, without putting too much strain on the knees and joints.

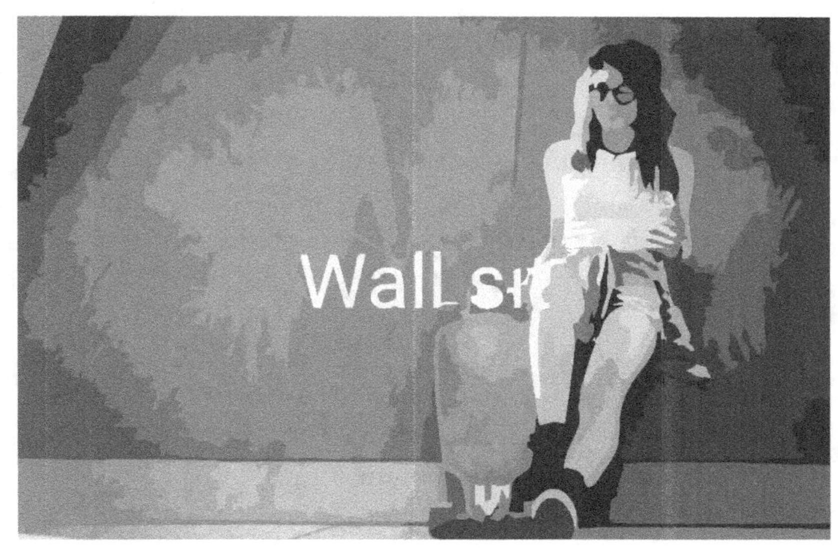

12. Supermans:

Supermans are a useful exercise for the lower back and for working the core. Lay on the ground face down with your legs straight and your arms overhead. Squeeze your glutes and lower back muscles at the peak of the movement as you simultaneously lift your arms, chest, and legs off the ground. Hold for a second before descending once more.

Supermans are advantageous for overall back health since they enhance lower back strength and posture.

14. Jump Rope:

Jumping rope is an enjoyable and efficient aerobic activity that burns a lot of calories quickly. Grab a jump rope, then begin leaping while keeping your feet together and rotating the rope with your wrists. Keep your attention on short, small hops to keep your beat steady.

Exercises with a jump rope increase agility, coordination, and cardiovascular endurance. They are a great option for workouts at home because they just require a modest amount of room and equipment.

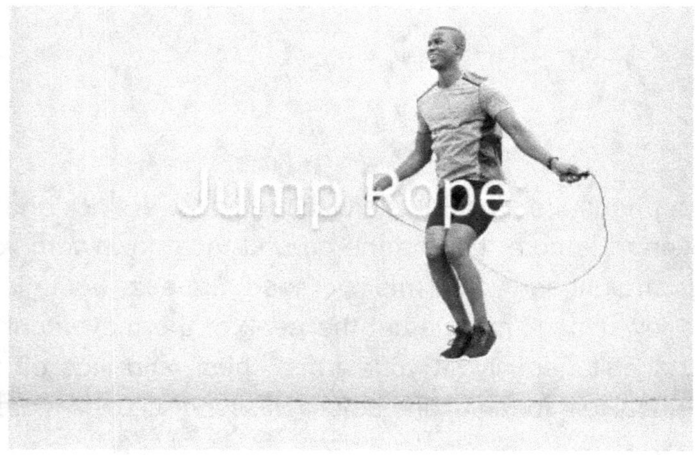

15. Donkey Kicks

Donkey kicks can be performed on all fours and primarily work the glutes. Begin on your hands and knees, placing your knees firmly beneath your hips and your hands directly behind your shoulders. Lift one leg up until the foot is facing the sky while maintaining a 90-degree bend in the knee. Before transferring to the second leg, bring your leg back down to the ground without letting it touch.

Donkey kicks are the best exercise for sculpting and strengthening the back because they effectively isolate and tone the glutes.

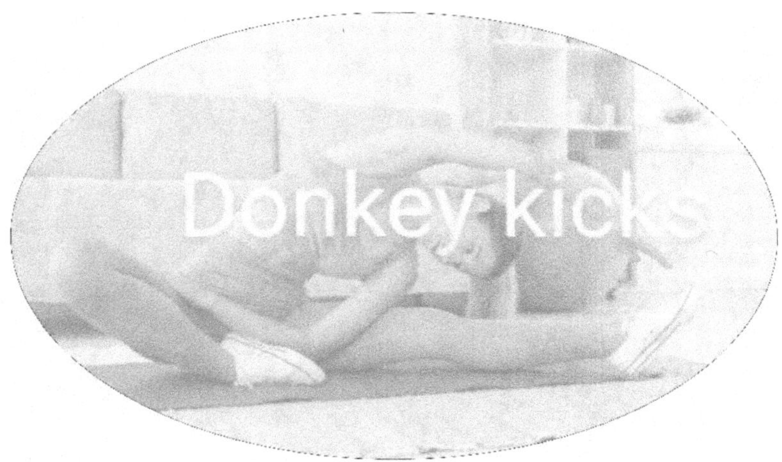

16. Side Lunges

Lunges on the side, sometimes referred to as lateral lunges, are great for working the inner and outer thighs. Standing with your feet together, step outward with your right foot while holding the left foot still.

By bending your right knee and pressing your hips back, you can lower your body as if you were sitting on a chair. Repeat on the other side, then go back to your starting position. Side lunges improve the flexibility and strength of the lower body, particularly the adductors and abductors.

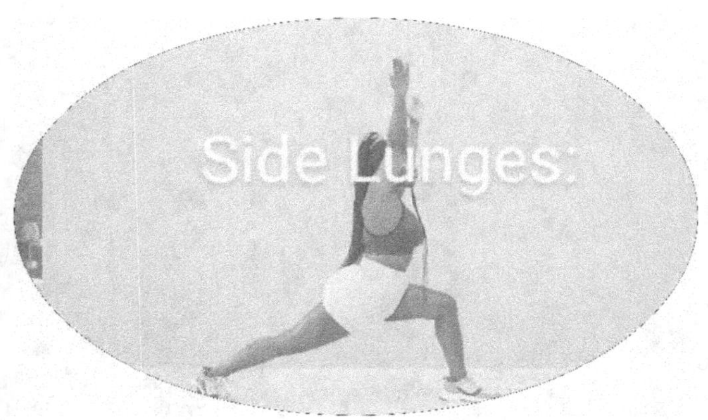

17. Inchworms

A dynamic stretching exercise that also works the core and shoulder muscles is called inchworms. Start off by assuming a hip-width stance.

Put your hands on the floor in front of you while bending at the waist. Reaching a plank position requires moving your hands forward while keeping your legs straight. Hold for a few moment, then revert to standing by moving your hands back toward your feet.

Inchworms bolster the core, mobilize the shoulder joints, and increase hamstring flexibility.

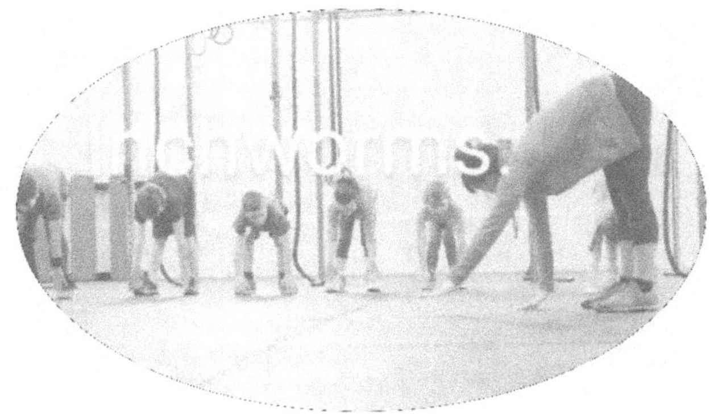

18. Side Plank

A version of the standard plank that targets the obliques and enhances balance and stability is the side plank. Begin by lying on your side with your legs stacked on top of one another and your elbow directly beneath your shoulder. Create a straight line from your head to your heels by lifting your hips off the floor. Hold this position for a predetermined period of time before switching to the opposite side.

Side planks tone the waistline by concentrating on the external obliques.

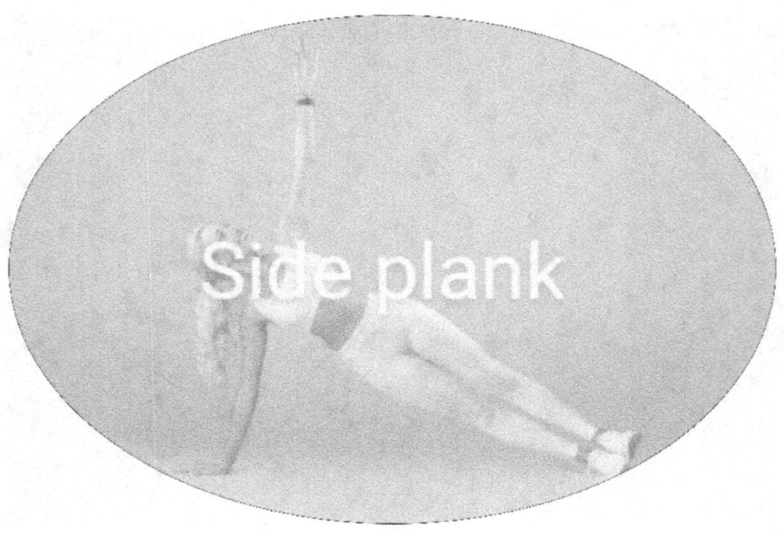

19. Glute Bridges:

Glute bridges work the hamstrings and core as well as the glutes and lower back. Legs bent and flat on the floor, hip-width apart, as you lay on your back. When your body is in a straight line from your shoulders to your knees, press through your heels to lift your hips off the ground. At the peak of the exercise, squeeze your glutes; then, lower yourself back down.

Glute bridges can help reduce lower back discomfort by strengthening the posterior chain.

20. Shadow Boxing:

Without a partner or equipment, shadow boxing is a workout with elements of boxing that involves throwing punches into the air. Assume a boxing stance while standing with your feet shoulder-width apart and your hands raised to shield your face. Alternate between jabs, crosses, hooks, and uppercuts as you deliver a succession of punches. Throughout the workout, maintain control over your movements and use your core.

Shadow boxing is a challenging cardio workout that enhances upper body strength, agility, and coordination.

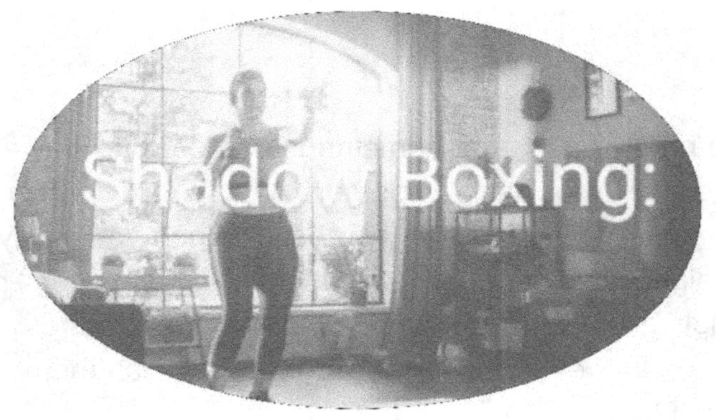

Incorporate these 20 home workouts for weight loss into your exercise routine, and remember to adjust the intensity and duration based on your fitness level. As with any exercise program, listen to your body, and consult a healthcare professional if you have any health concerns or medical conditions. Consistency and dedication will lead to progress, helping you achieve your weight loss and fitness goals.

CONCLUSION

We've discovered the secret to self-transformation through the world of at-home workouts for weight loss in the intriguing pages of this book. We've learned from working through the 20 dynamic exercises that real transformation starts within of us. Each workout is a profound voyage of self-discovery and empowerment, representing more than simply physical movement.

We've discovered that being fit is about embracing our power, resilience, and potential rather than just losing weight or gaining muscle. Although the road to change is not always easy, we have learned the power to overcome challenges and emerge even more powerful than before through tenacity and self-compassion.

We accept the notion that we are not limited by constraints but rather by the tales we decide to believe as we move into the rhythm of change. We have discovered a deeper connection between mind and body—a union that feeds our growth and equips us to meet life's difficulties with unshakable courage—by rewriting those tales and lighting our inner fire.

We have been motivated to embrace our weaknesses and celebrate our successes by reading these pages. As we continue on our path of self-discovery, we are encouraged to shine brightly and encourage others to embrace their own development.

So, as you put this book away, keep in mind that you have the ability to change. Accept your individuality, rejoice in your accomplishments, and remember that the road has only just begun. Embody the power, authenticity, and self-assurance that have been sparked throughout this journey, and allow it lead you to a life of limitless potential.

Go ahead and start your journey toward self-transformation now. The brilliance of your genuine self is what the world awaits. Accept change, accept development, and acknowledge the incredible power you possess.

This plan includes a variety of nutritious and delicious recipes to help you achieve your weight loss goals. Remember to consult with a healthcare professional or a registered dietitian before starting any new diet or weight loss plan.

Day 1:

Greek yogurt for breakfast, topped with berries and almonds.

Lunch: Mixed green salad with grilled chicken breast and vinaigrette. Dinner will be baked salmon with quinoa and steam broccoli.

Day 2:

Breakfast: Whole-grain toast and a veggie omelet (with spinach, bell peppers, and onions).

Lunch: Whole-grain tortilla wrap with turkey and avocado.

Dinner will be tofu stir-fried with a variety of vegetables and brown rice.

Day 3:

Breakfast is overnight oats with almond milk, chopped fruit, and chia seeds.

Lunch will be a quinoa salad with feta cheese, cucumber, cherry tomatoes, and lemon dressing. Dinner will be roasted sweet potatoes and asparagus with baked chicken thighs.

Day 4:

Breakfast: Cottage cheese topped with honey and sliced peaches.

Lunch will be grilled shrimp over zucchini noodles with pesto.

Dinner will be stuffed bell peppers with cauliflower rice and lean ground turkey.

Day 5:

Smoothie for breakfast made with banana, spinach, almond milk, and protein powder.

Lunch will be lentil soup and a mixed green salad.

Dinner will be baked cod with wild rice and Brussels sprouts.

Day 6:

Breakfast will consist of whole-grain pancakes, Greek yogurt, and fresh fruit.
Chickpea and vegetable curry for lunch.
Dinner will be grilled steak with sautéed mushrooms and spinach on the side.

Day 7:

Breakfast toast with avocado, cherry tomatoes, and poached eggs.
Lunch will be a mixed greens salad with tuna and a lemon-tahini dressing. Dinner will be baked eggplant parmesan with green beans on the side.

Week 2, 3, and 4:

Repeat the meal plan from Week 1 or mix and match the recipes to keep the variety while staying within your caloric and nutritional needs.

Drink plenty of water throughout the day to stay hydrated, and think about having nutritious snacks between meals such Greek yogurt, almonds, or fruits.

To lose weight, keep in mind that portion management and regular exercise are equally crucial. Change the meal plan to suit your nutritional needs, food sensitivities, and specific weight reduction objectives.

We sincerely appreciate you reading "Transform Within: Embrace the Journey of Self-Discovery and Empowerment" and starting this transforming journey with us. It has been a gift to you as well as to the authors of this book that you chose to read its pages.

We wish you continued success as a result of the lessons, activities, and inspiring words offered in these pages. You opened the door to self-discovery and personal improvement as you embraced the world of at-home workouts for weight loss.

.

We are grateful to have been a part of your route because we are inspired by your dedication to this transformational journey. May the lessons you've learned here serve as a guide as you continue to discover your inner strength, accept who you are, and realize your full potential.

Keep in mind that this book is merely a starting point for your road to a more powerful and meaningful life. Have faith in your ability to make great changes in your life and the lives of others around you as you move forward.

Finally, we would want to express our sincere gratitude for picking "Transform Within" to travel with you on this wonderful journey. We have faith in your ability to succeed in anything you set your mind to. Continue shining brightly and serving as an inspiration to others.

With sincere appreciation,

[HARRY LANCE]

WORKOUT LOG

NAME:___________________________   GOALS:___________________________

EXERCISES	SETS	REPS	WT	REST	TIME	1 RM	NOTES

DATE:__________   WEIGHT:__________   SLEEP:__________   CALORIES:__________

EXERCISES	SETS	REPS	WT	REST	TIME	1 RM	NOTES

DATE:__________   WEIGHT:__________   SLEEP:__________   CALORIES:__________

EXERCISES	SETS	REPS	WT	REST	TIME	1 RM	NOTES

DATE:__________   WEIGHT:__________   SLEEP:__________   CALORIES:__________

EXERCISES	SETS	REPS	WT	REST	TIME	1 RM	NOTES

DATE:__________   WEIGHT:__________   SLEEP:__________   CALORIES:__________

EXERCISES	SETS	REPS	WT	REST	TIME	1 RM	NOTES

DATE:__________   WEIGHT:__________   SLEEP:__________   CALORIES:__________

WORKOUT LOG

NAME:________________________ GOALS:_______________________

EXERCISES	SETS	REPS	WT	REST	TIME	1 RM	NOTES

DATE:__________ WEIGHT:__________ SLEEP:__________ CALORIES:__________

EXERCISES	SETS	REPS	WT	REST	TIME	1 RM	NOTES

DATE:__________ WEIGHT:__________ SLEEP:__________ CALORIES:__________

EXERCISES	SETS	REPS	WT	REST	TIME	1 RM	NOTES

DATE:__________ WEIGHT:__________ SLEEP:__________ CALORIES:__________

EXERCISES	SETS	REPS	WT	REST	TIME	1 RM	NOTES

DATE:__________ WEIGHT:__________ SLEEP:__________ CALORIES:__________

EXERCISES	SETS	REPS	WT	REST	TIME	1 RM	NOTES

DATE:__________ WEIGHT:__________ SLEEP:__________ CALORIES:__________

WORKOUT LOG

NAME:________________________   GOALS:________________________

EXERCISES	SETS	REPS	WT	REST	TIME	1 RM	NOTES

DATE:__________   WEIGHT:__________   SLEEP:__________   CALORIES:__________

EXERCISES	SETS	REPS	WT	REST	TIME	1 RM	NOTES

DATE:__________   WEIGHT:__________   SLEEP:__________   CALORIES:__________

EXERCISES	SETS	REPS	WT	REST	TIME	1 RM	NOTES

DATE:__________   WEIGHT:__________   SLEEP:__________   CALORIES:__________

EXERCISES	SETS	REPS	WT	REST	TIME	1 RM	NOTES

DATE:__________   WEIGHT:__________   SLEEP:__________   CALORIES:__________

EXERCISES	SETS	REPS	WT	REST	TIME	1 RM	NOTES

DATE:__________   WEIGHT:__________   SLEEP:__________   CALORIES:__________

WORKOUT LOG

NAME:_______________________ GOALS:_______________________

EXERCISES	SETS	REPS	WT	REST	TIME	1 RM	NOTES

DATE:__________ WEIGHT:__________ SLEEP:__________ CALORIES:__________

EXERCISES	SETS	REPS	WT	REST	TIME	1 RM	NOTES

DATE:__________ WEIGHT:__________ SLEEP:__________ CALORIES:__________

EXERCISES	SETS	REPS	WT	REST	TIME	1 RM	NOTES

DATE:__________ WEIGHT:__________ SLEEP:__________ CALORIES:__________

EXERCISES	SETS	REPS	WT	REST	TIME	1 RM	NOTES

DATE:__________ WEIGHT:__________ SLEEP:__________ CALORIES:__________

EXERCISES	SETS	REPS	WT	REST	TIME	1 RM	NOTES

DATE:__________ WEIGHT:__________ SLEEP:__________ CALORIES:__________

WORKOUT LOG

NAME:________________________   GOALS:____________________

EXERCISES	SETS	REPS	WT	REST	TIME	1 RM	NOTES

DATE:__________   WEIGHT:__________   SLEEP:__________   CALORIES:__________

EXERCISES	SETS	REPS	WT	REST	TIME	1 RM	NOTES

DATE:__________   WEIGHT:__________   SLEEP:__________   CALORIES:__________

EXERCISES	SETS	REPS	WT	REST	TIME	1 RM	NOTES

DATE:__________   WEIGHT:__________   SLEEP:__________   CALORIES:__________

EXERCISES	SETS	REPS	WT	REST	TIME	1 RM	NOTES

DATE:__________   WEIGHT:__________   SLEEP:__________   CALORIES:__________

EXERCISES	SETS	REPS	WT	REST	TIME	1 RM	NOTES

DATE:__________   WEIGHT:__________   SLEEP:__________   CALORIES:__________

WORKOUT LOG

NAME:________________________ GOALS:________________________

EXERCISES	SETS	REPS	WT	REST	TIME	1 RM	NOTES

DATE:__________ WEIGHT:__________ SLEEP:__________ CALORIES:__________

EXERCISES	SETS	REPS	WT	REST	TIME	1 RM	NOTES

DATE:__________ WEIGHT:__________ SLEEP:__________ CALORIES:__________

EXERCISES	SETS	REPS	WT	REST	TIME	1 RM	NOTES

DATE:__________ WEIGHT:__________ SLEEP:__________ CALORIES:__________

EXERCISES	SETS	REPS	WT	REST	TIME	1 RM	NOTES

DATE:__________ WEIGHT:__________ SLEEP:__________ CALORIES:__________

EXERCISES	SETS	REPS	WT	REST	TIME	1 RM	NOTES

DATE:__________ WEIGHT:__________ SLEEP:__________ CALORIES:__________

WORKOUT LOG

NAME:__________________________ GOALS:__________________________

EXERCISES	SETS	REPS	WT	REST	TIME	1 RM	NOTES

DATE:__________ WEIGHT:__________ SLEEP:__________ CALORIES:__________

EXERCISES	SETS	REPS	WT	REST	TIME	1 RM	NOTES

DATE:__________ WEIGHT:__________ SLEEP:__________ CALORIES:__________

EXERCISES	SETS	REPS	WT	REST	TIME	1 RM	NOTES

DATE:__________ WEIGHT:__________ SLEEP:__________ CALORIES:__________

EXERCISES	SETS	REPS	WT	REST	TIME	1 RM	NOTES

DATE:__________ WEIGHT:__________ SLEEP:__________ CALORIES:__________

EXERCISES	SETS	REPS	WT	REST	TIME	1 RM	NOTES

DATE:__________ WEIGHT:__________ SLEEP:__________ CALORIES:__________

WORKOUT LOG

NAME:_________________________ GOALS:_____________________

EXERCISES	SETS	REPS	WT	REST	TIME	1 RM	NOTES

DATE:__________   WEIGHT:__________   SLEEP:__________   CALORIES:__________

EXERCISES	SETS	REPS	WT	REST	TIME	1 RM	NOTES

DATE:__________   WEIGHT:__________   SLEEP:__________   CALORIES:__________

EXERCISES	SETS	REPS	WT	REST	TIME	1 RM	NOTES

DATE:__________   WEIGHT:__________   SLEEP:__________   CALORIES:__________

EXERCISES	SETS	REPS	WT	REST	TIME	1 RM	NOTES

DATE:__________   WEIGHT:__________   SLEEP:__________   CALORIES:__________

EXERCISES	SETS	REPS	WT	REST	TIME	1 RM	NOTES

DATE:__________   WEIGHT:__________   SLEEP:__________   CALORIES:__________

WORKOUT LOG

NAME:____________________   GOALS:____________________

EXERCISES	SETS	REPS	WT	REST	TIME	1 RM	NOTES

DATE:__________   WEIGHT:__________   SLEEP:__________   CALORIES:__________

EXERCISES	SETS	REPS	WT	REST	TIME	1 RM	NOTES

DATE:__________   WEIGHT:__________   SLEEP:__________   CALORIES:__________

EXERCISES	SETS	REPS	WT	REST	TIME	1 RM	NOTES

DATE:__________   WEIGHT:__________   SLEEP:__________   CALORIES:__________

EXERCISES	SETS	REPS	WT	REST	TIME	1 RM	NOTES

DATE:__________   WEIGHT:__________   SLEEP:__________   CALORIES:__________

EXERCISES	SETS	REPS	WT	REST	TIME	1 RM	NOTES

DATE:__________   WEIGHT:__________   SLEEP:__________   CALORIES:__________

WORKOUT LOG

NAME:_______________________   GOALS:_______________________

EXERCISES	SETS	REPS	WT	REST	TIME	1 RM	NOTES

DATE:_________   WEIGHT:_________   SLEEP:_________   CALORIES:_________

EXERCISES	SETS	REPS	WT	REST	TIME	1 RM	NOTES

DATE:_________   WEIGHT:_________   SLEEP:_________   CALORIES:_________

EXERCISES	SETS	REPS	WT	REST	TIME	1 RM	NOTES

DATE:_________   WEIGHT:_________   SLEEP:_________   CALORIES:_________

EXERCISES	SETS	REPS	WT	REST	TIME	1 RM	NOTES

DATE:_________   WEIGHT:_________   SLEEP:_________   CALORIES:_________

EXERCISES	SETS	REPS	WT	REST	TIME	1 RM	NOTES

DATE:_________   WEIGHT:_________   SLEEP:_________   CALORIES:_________

WORKOUT LOG

NAME:________________________ GOALS:________________________

EXERCISES	SETS	REPS	WT	REST	TIME	1 RM	NOTES

DATE:__________ WEIGHT:__________ SLEEP:__________ CALORIES:__________

EXERCISES	SETS	REPS	WT	REST	TIME	1 RM	NOTES

DATE:__________ WEIGHT:__________ SLEEP:__________ CALORIES:__________

EXERCISES	SETS	REPS	WT	REST	TIME	1 RM	NOTES

DATE:__________ WEIGHT:__________ SLEEP:__________ CALORIES:__________

EXERCISES	SETS	REPS	WT	REST	TIME	1 RM	NOTES

DATE:__________ WEIGHT:__________ SLEEP:__________ CALORIES:__________

EXERCISES	SETS	REPS	WT	REST	TIME	1 RM	NOTES

DATE:__________ WEIGHT:__________ SLEEP:__________ CALORIES:__________

WORKOUT LOG

NAME:_________________________   GOALS:_____________________

EXERCISES	SETS	REPS	WT	REST	TIME	1 RM	NOTES

DATE:__________   WEIGHT:__________   SLEEP:__________   CALORIES:__________

EXERCISES	SETS	REPS	WT	REST	TIME	1 RM	NOTES

DATE:__________   WEIGHT:__________   SLEEP:__________   CALORIES:__________

EXERCISES	SETS	REPS	WT	REST	TIME	1 RM	NOTES

DATE:__________   WEIGHT:__________   SLEEP:__________   CALORIES:__________

EXERCISES	SETS	REPS	WT	REST	TIME	1 RM	NOTES

DATE:__________   WEIGHT:__________   SLEEP:__________   CALORIES:__________

EXERCISES	SETS	REPS	WT	REST	TIME	1 RM	NOTES

DATE:__________   WEIGHT:__________   SLEEP:__________   CALORIES:__________

WORKOUT LOG

NAME:_________________________   GOALS:_________________________

EXERCISES	SETS	REPS	WT	REST	TIME	1 RM	NOTES

DATE:__________   WEIGHT:__________   SLEEP:__________   CALORIES:__________

EXERCISES	SETS	REPS	WT	REST	TIME	1 RM	NOTES

DATE:__________   WEIGHT:__________   SLEEP:__________   CALORIES:__________

EXERCISES	SETS	REPS	WT	REST	TIME	1 RM	NOTES

DATE:__________   WEIGHT:__________   SLEEP:__________   CALORIES:__________

EXERCISES	SETS	REPS	WT	REST	TIME	1 RM	NOTES

DATE:__________   WEIGHT:__________   SLEEP:__________   CALORIES:__________

EXERCISES	SETS	REPS	WT	REST	TIME	1 RM	NOTES

DATE:__________   WEIGHT:__________   SLEEP:__________   CALORIES:__________

WORKOUT LOG

NAME:____________________________ GOALS:____________________________

EXERCISES	SETS	REPS	WT	REST	TIME	1 RM	NOTES

DATE:__________ WEIGHT:__________ SLEEP:__________ CALORIES:__________

EXERCISES	SETS	REPS	WT	REST	TIME	1 RM	NOTES

DATE:__________ WEIGHT:__________ SLEEP:__________ CALORIES:__________

EXERCISES	SETS	REPS	WT	REST	TIME	1 RM	NOTES

DATE:__________ WEIGHT:__________ SLEEP:__________ CALORIES:__________

EXERCISES	SETS	REPS	WT	REST	TIME	1 RM	NOTES

DATE:__________ WEIGHT:__________ SLEEP:__________ CALORIES:__________

EXERCISES	SETS	REPS	WT	REST	TIME	1 RM	NOTES

DATE:__________ WEIGHT:__________ SLEEP:__________ CALORIES:__________

WORKOUT LOG

NAME:_________________________ GOALS:_________________________

EXERCISES	SETS	REPS	WT	REST	TIME	1 RM	NOTES

DATE:__________   WEIGHT:__________   SLEEP:__________   CALORIES:__________

EXERCISES	SETS	REPS	WT	REST	TIME	1 RM	NOTES

DATE:__________   WEIGHT:__________   SLEEP:__________   CALORIES:__________

EXERCISES	SETS	REPS	WT	REST	TIME	1 RM	NOTES

DATE:__________   WEIGHT:__________   SLEEP:__________   CALORIES:__________

EXERCISES	SETS	REPS	WT	REST	TIME	1 RM	NOTES

DATE:__________   WEIGHT:__________   SLEEP:__________   CALORIES:__________

EXERCISES	SETS	REPS	WT	REST	TIME	1 RM	NOTES

DATE:__________   WEIGHT:__________   SLEEP:__________   CALORIES:__________

WORKOUT LOG

NAME:___________________________   GOALS:___________________________

EXERCISES	SETS	REPS	WT	REST	TIME	1 RM	NOTES

DATE:__________   WEIGHT:__________   SLEEP:__________   CALORIES:__________

EXERCISES	SETS	REPS	WT	REST	TIME	1 RM	NOTES

DATE:__________   WEIGHT:__________   SLEEP:__________   CALORIES:__________

EXERCISES	SETS	REPS	WT	REST	TIME	1 RM	NOTES

DATE:__________   WEIGHT:__________   SLEEP:__________   CALORIES:__________

EXERCISES	SETS	REPS	WT	REST	TIME	1 RM	NOTES

DATE:__________   WEIGHT:__________   SLEEP:__________   CALORIES:__________

EXERCISES	SETS	REPS	WT	REST	TIME	1 RM	NOTES

DATE:__________   WEIGHT:__________   SLEEP:__________   CALORIES:__________

WORKOUT LOG

NAME:_________________________   GOALS:_________________________

EXERCISES	SETS	REPS	WT	REST	TIME	1 RM	NOTES

DATE:___________   WEIGHT:__________   SLEEP:__________   CALORIES:__________

EXERCISES	SETS	REPS	WT	REST	TIME	1 RM	NOTES

DATE:___________   WEIGHT:__________   SLEEP:__________   CALORIES:__________

EXERCISES	SETS	REPS	WT	REST	TIME	1 RM	NOTES

DATE:___________   WEIGHT:__________   SLEEP:__________   CALORIES:__________

EXERCISES	SETS	REPS	WT	REST	TIME	1 RM	NOTES

DATE:___________   WEIGHT:__________   SLEEP:__________   CALORIES:__________

EXERCISES	SETS	REPS	WT	REST	TIME	1 RM	NOTES

DATE:___________   WEIGHT:__________   SLEEP:__________   CALORIES:__________

WORKOUT LOG

NAME:_________________________   GOALS:_________________________

EXERCISES	SETS	REPS	WT	REST	TIME	1 RM	NOTES

DATE:_________   WEIGHT:_________   SLEEP:_________   CALORIES:_________

EXERCISES	SETS	REPS	WT	REST	TIME	1 RM	NOTES

DATE:_________   WEIGHT:_________   SLEEP:_________   CALORIES:_________

EXERCISES	SETS	REPS	WT	REST	TIME	1 RM	NOTES

DATE:_________   WEIGHT:_________   SLEEP:_________   CALORIES:_________

EXERCISES	SETS	REPS	WT	REST	TIME	1 RM	NOTES

DATE:_________   WEIGHT:_________   SLEEP:_________   CALORIES:_________

EXERCISES	SETS	REPS	WT	REST	TIME	1 RM	NOTES

DATE:_________   WEIGHT:_________   SLEEP:_________   CALORIES:_________

WORKOUT LOG

NAME:________________________   GOALS:________________________

EXERCISES	SETS	REPS	WT	REST	TIME	1 RM	NOTES

DATE:__________   WEIGHT:__________   SLEEP:__________   CALORIES:__________

EXERCISES	SETS	REPS	WT	REST	TIME	1 RM	NOTES

DATE:__________   WEIGHT:__________   SLEEP:__________   CALORIES:__________

EXERCISES	SETS	REPS	WT	REST	TIME	1 RM	NOTES

DATE:__________   WEIGHT:__________   SLEEP:__________   CALORIES:__________

EXERCISES	SETS	REPS	WT	REST	TIME	1 RM	NOTES

DATE:__________   WEIGHT:__________   SLEEP:__________   CALORIES:__________

EXERCISES	SETS	REPS	WT	REST	TIME	1 RM	NOTES

DATE:__________   WEIGHT:__________   SLEEP:__________   CALORIES:__________

WORKOUT LOG

NAME:________________________   GOALS:________________________

EXERCISES	SETS	REPS	WT	REST	TIME	1 RM	NOTES

DATE:_________   WEIGHT:_________   SLEEP:_________   CALORIES:_________

EXERCISES	SETS	REPS	WT	REST	TIME	1 RM	NOTES

DATE:_________   WEIGHT:_________   SLEEP:_________   CALORIES:_________

EXERCISES	SETS	REPS	WT	REST	TIME	1 RM	NOTES

DATE:_________   WEIGHT:_________   SLEEP:_________   CALORIES:_________

EXERCISES	SETS	REPS	WT	REST	TIME	1 RM	NOTES

DATE:_________   WEIGHT:_________   SLEEP:_________   CALORIES:_________

EXERCISES	SETS	REPS	WT	REST	TIME	1 RM	NOTES

DATE:_________   WEIGHT:_________   SLEEP:_________   CALORIES:_________

www.ingramcontent.com/pod-product-compliance
Lightning Source LLC
Chambersburg PA
CBHW071116260726
48661CB00006B/2625